MEZZA
STYLE GUIDE

MEZZA

STYLE GUIDE

A Holistic Lifestyle Guide for the Woman over 45

Jacqueline Grund

BOOKLOGIX®
Alpharetta, GA

ISBN: 978-1-6653-0265-4 - Paperback

ISBN: 978-1-6653-0298-2 - Hardcover

Printed in the United States of America   0 9 1 4 2 1

⊗This paper meets the requirements of ANSI/NISO Z39.48-1992 (Permanence of Paper)

Cover Art by Lindsey Kate Fashion Illustration and Design, www.lindsey-kate.com

To my parents, who believed in me.

To my husband, who loves me.

To my kids and grandkids, whom I adore.

Make this style guide yours

by filling in your own words as you read!

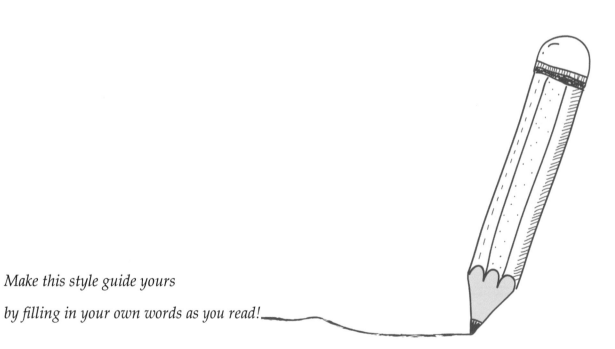

INTRODUCTION
Why a style guide?

There have been many books written about style and fashion throughout the ages. This one is different. As an extension of our digital online fashion and lifestyle platform, the *Mezza Style Guide* aims to be a strategic way to highlight not only the outer beauty of women over the age of forty-five but the inner beauty as well. The goal is that this is not only a guide for women, but a physical representation that there is life, and style, after forty-five, you just have to know how to take ownership of it!

I have spent the greater part of my adult years in the crazy world of fashion, and I wouldn't have it any other way. I was introduced to style at a young age from my mother, Sylvia, to my oh-so-stylish grandmother and all of my aunts and great aunts who came before me who represented fashion so well. What this taught me was that style wasn't just about what you wore but about how you feel when expressing yourself through fashion. I've dedicated this guide to all of the women in their middle years. The kids are all grown up and you can be YOU again! So, what will you do with your power?

I am here to tell you that the second half of your life is just beginning and your Mezza family is with you every step of the way!

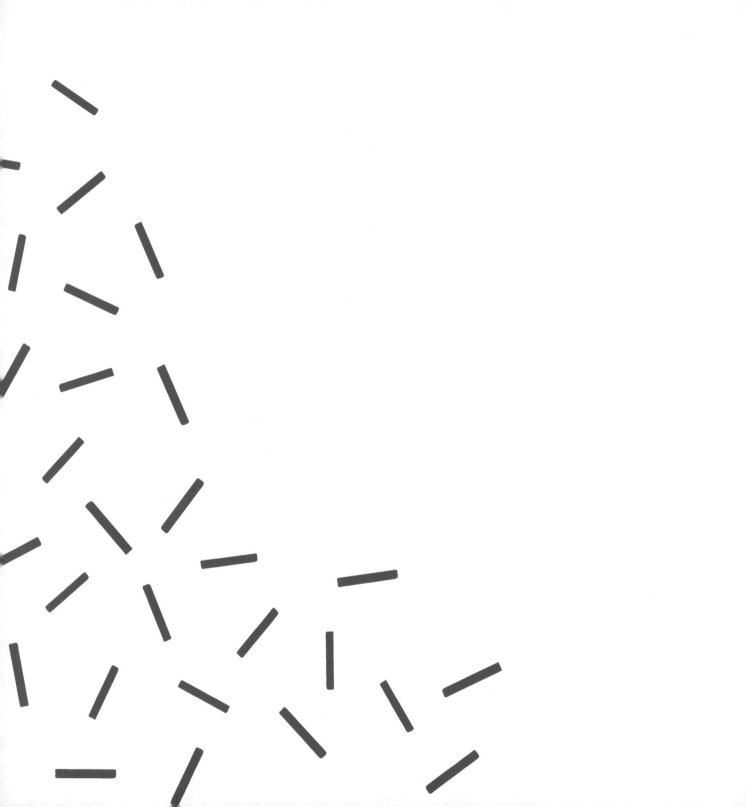

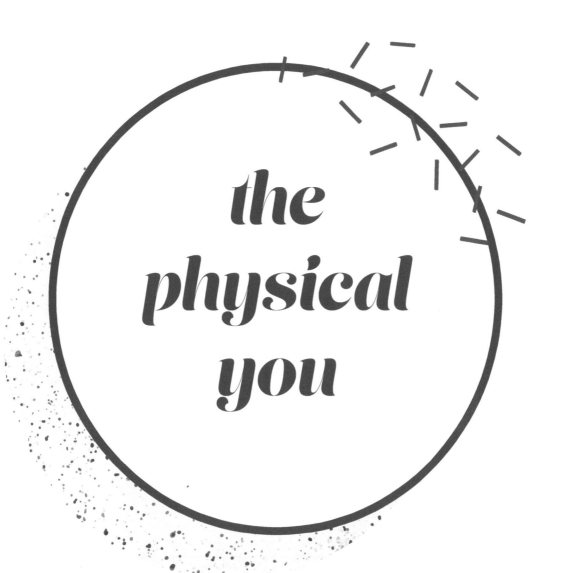

the
physical
you

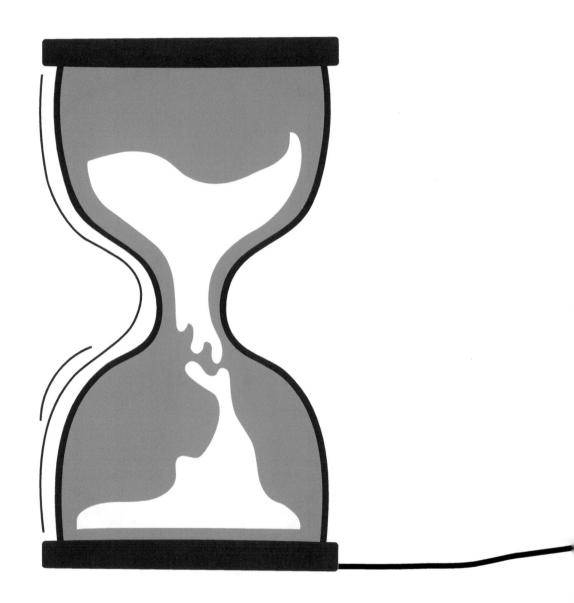

You're yelling, tired, grumpy, sleepy, and not really loving *you* so much. It's happening. You are now peri- or postmenopausal. So, what now?

Ladies, life doesn't just stop when your period does. You are still you, so BE YOU! Sometimes, finding the way back to who you are in this stage of life can be difficult. That's okay. Our minds can psych us out of a fulfilling life if we keep putting age limits on everything that we do. Just because you've entered the second half of your life doesn't mean you don't get a chance to be the healthiest *you* that you can be. Health isn't just for our younger selves; we have to maintain it as we progress through life. You're only as young as you feel, so why not feel the best?

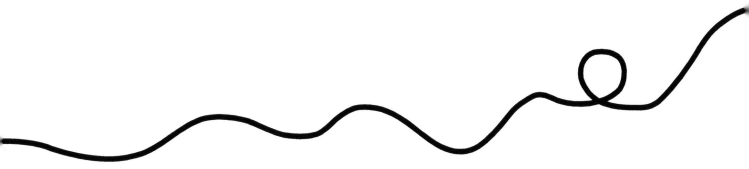

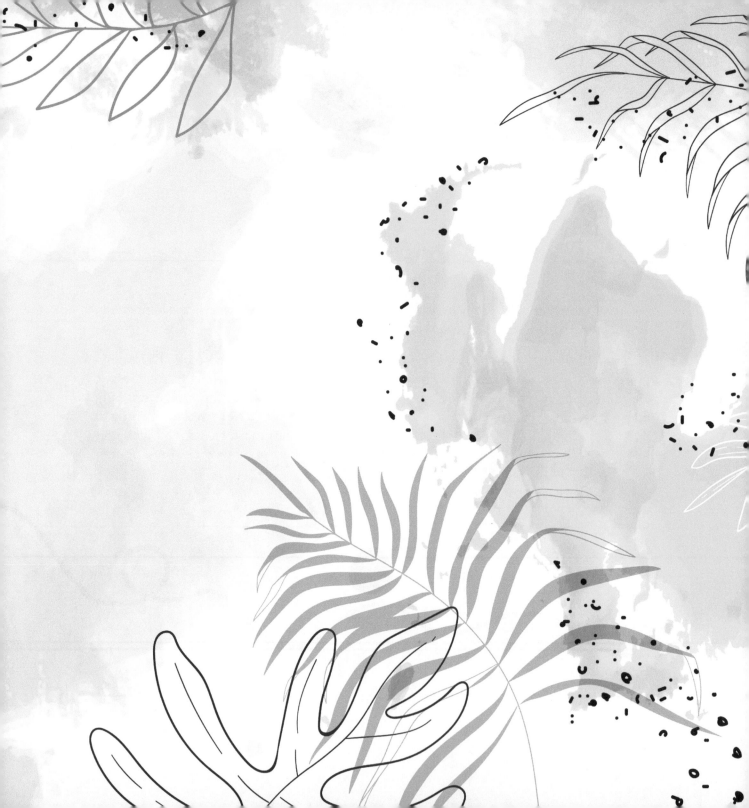

HOLISTIC HEALTH

We all want a way to subside the harrowing effects of menopause. One of the most beneficial things you can do for yourself is to do what you can to start *feeling* like yourself again. One way to start feeling your best is to start researching holistic approaches to hormone management.

By definition, holistic medicine and health is a health practice that takes into consideration the whole person through mind, body, spirit, and emotions in order to gain the most optimal level of overall wellness. The ultimate goal is to gain the "proper balance in life"!

Basically, holistic medicine practitioners believe that everything in the body is interconnected. Therefore, when one part of the body has an imbalance, such as your hormones, it can have an effect on other parts of the body—thus holistic medicine may be able to provide a solution to those hot flashes!

AVOID THE TRIGGERS

Did you know that there are foods that can actually trigger symptoms of menopause? Things like caffeine, alcoholic drinks, and spicy and sugary foods are common triggers for hot flashes, night sweats, and mood swings. If you want a way to find out if specific foods or drinks trigger your symptoms, try keeping a "Symptom Diary." By writing down when you've reacted to certain foods, you can begin to take back control of your life!

NATURAL SUPPLEMENTS

Mother Nature also has her way of gaining control over menopause. Herbal supplements such as black cohosh, red clover, ginseng, and kava, to name a few, have natural elements that reduce the appearance of symptoms, including hot flashes, sleep disturbances, or just make women feel better overall. Though we always think natural is best, it is good to note that any natural or herbal supplement should be used with caution, as many of these therapies are not as closely regulated as regular medically prescribed drugs. Always refer to your healthcare provider when considering this form of therapy.

HEALTHY LIFESTYLE

It's okay to avoid certain foods, but like with everything else, maintaining an overall healthy lifestyle will reduce your risk of getting any symptoms at all. A lifestyle encompasses every area of your life from the foods you eat and drink to your level of physical activity to even your emotional wellness. Keeping your diet clean, exercising regularly, and keeping yourself happy and motivated all make a difference in your menopausal journey. Don't forget to drink the correct amount of water for you!

CALCIUM & VITAMIN D

Menopause can take a heavy hit on our bones, so eating foods that are rich in calcium—like yogurt, milk, or cheese—are good for bone health, which can be a benefit to us ladies who may develop osteoporosis. Healthy sources of vitamin D can also lower the risk of developing hip issues due to bone weakness. A healthy dose of calcium can also be found in cereals, milk alternatives, and fruit juices for my ladies who want to avoid dairy. Leafy veggies like spinach, kale, and collard greens will also get the job done.

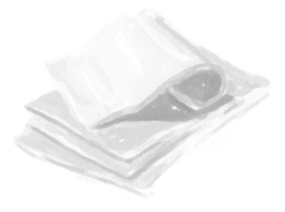

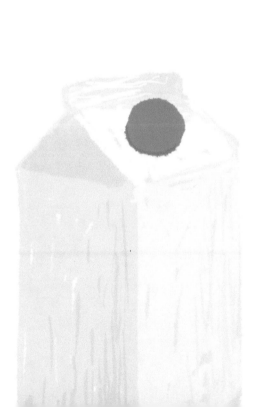

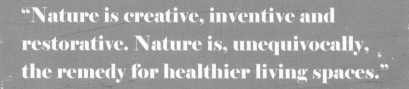

"Nature is creative, inventive and restorative. Nature is, unequivocally, the remedy for healthier living spaces."

—JOHANNE MORIN,
Home Décor and Feng Shui contributor
for the *Mezza Reviews* blog

WEIGHT

It's common that as we age, extra weight can just "appear" out of nowhere! Whether it's from out-of-balance hormones, lifestyle, or even genetics, as we age, our weight tends to fluctuate the most. Keep the body fat to a minimum—especially around that waist area—to decrease the chances of developing heart disease or diabetes. If you can lose at least 10 percent of body fat you just might eliminate those hot flashes and night sweats altogether. Now, wouldn't that be a dream?

WATCHING YOUR WEIGHT

Today, there are many options for people who need a little extra motivation to shed unwanted pounds and inspire healthy living to promote overall wellness.

A program we are all familiar with, which uses points, assigns every food and beverage a point value, based on its nutrition, and leverages details about food preferences and lifestyle to match each member to one of three comprehensive ways to follow the program. As a member, you'll also have access to expert-led workshops to provide practical tools and behavior change techniques to help you in your journey along the way. I have used this program, and I continue to do so through the ease of my phone.

WORKING OUT AT HOME

It's safe to say that working out from home is here to stay due to our current state of our society post pandemic. From videos, to bikes, to treadmill machines, and online workouts. This is a safe and healthy trend for people in the middle of their life who have underlying health issues and who don't feel comfortable at large gyms.

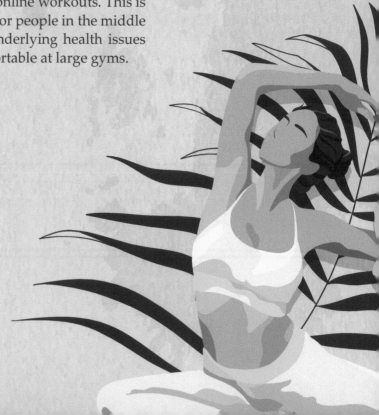

PHYSICAL HEALTH

Some women think that when you turn forty-five, and beyond, it's all of a sudden a death sentence; almost like there's now a countdown to their lives. This is not true! At forty-five, it's time for an all-new chapter of life and beyond. It is the starting point for the rest of your life, as long as you're able to embrace it.

"You have to take care of yourself, your body, your mind, take care of your soul—be your own keeper." —Jennifer Lopez

True words from Jennifer Lopez, who is in her fifties—Wow! While we may not all look like Jennifer Lopez, we can take note and continue to reinvent ourselves for as long as we wish. In order to do that, physicality for us is important. If you don't use it, you'll lose it! The more we keep our bodies moving and keep our bones and joints strong, the healthier we'll be and the more confident we can remain.

After forty-five, our metabolism needs our attention! This is what plays a part in our weight management, hormone balance, even our emotional well-being. If we can aim for a little bit of moderate exercise every week, I think we'll be in good shape—pun intended!

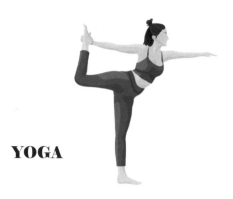

YOGA

"Yoga is a mirror to look at ourselves from within." —B. K. S. Iyengar

While yoga is a trend for the younger crowd, it's a time for moving inward for us ladies over the age of forty-five. Yoga International, to my understanding, described vedic philosophy as being "the first twenty-five years of our lives are meant for study, the second twenty-five years are a time for family and world achievements, the third twenty-five years is the time to move inward, and the last twenty-five years is meant for us to become the teachers."

While this philosophy promotes our youthful energy being reserved for our first twenty-five years, I say let our youthful energy speak for itself at any age! No matter if you're a first-timer or a well-versed yogi, the art of yoga can not only be a great practice for maintaining flexibility and strength in our muscles and joints, but can also become a great hobby for us empty nesters. Don't be afraid of starting a new hobby like yoga. You can gain better sleep habits, less chronic pain, and you'll even be able to move a little better. Not to mention your doctor will love you for it! Just make sure you sign up for a class or program that caters to your needs if you have any physical limitations.

A little practice goes a long way so commit to just ten to twenty minutes a day and watch the transformation you'll feel inside!

PILATES

"Change happens through movement, and movement heals." —Joseph Pilates

Now, many think Pilates is reserved for the young, athletic people . . . wrong! Done correctly, Pilates actually doesn't take a heavy toll on the body for women over forty-five or put unnecessary strain on the heart, which is a recipe for success!

What makes Pilates a go-to for some women is that it is a complete mind-body workout; it involves concentrating on your flowy movements while practicing quality exercises that puts a focus on the core. Your core is the central part of your body and is important to keep strong as we age. Good core muscles allow you to maintain good posture and can help keep your pelvis and shoulder muscles aligned with the rest of your body.

Pilates can actually be considered *anti-aging*! Similar to yoga though, you have to find what will work for you. Signing up for the intermediate class when you are beginning may not make your body love you. For those of us wanting to keep living life to the fullest with strong and lean muscles, Pilates is just the beginning!

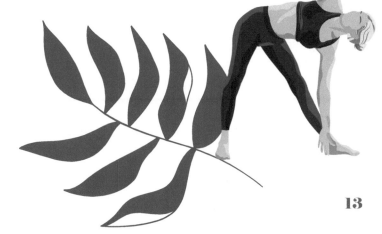

BARRE

"Don't wait for the right opportunity: create it." —George Bernard Shaw

For some of us, we have had to give up some of the exercise classes that we have enjoyed throughout the years, such as aerobics, high-impact exercises, and maybe even athletic training. While barre may provide a little more struggle in the beginning to get comfortable with, the results can be lasting and beneficial.

Barre exercise classes can take us out of our comfort zone and allow us to have different options for different body types in exercise. Barre classes tone your muscles and sculpt your body in ways that you may not realize would be possible over the age of forty-five. The classes can fit a range of generations of women and get the body moving in ways that benefit the overall health of the body.

WALKING

"If you get tired, learn to rest, not quit." —Banksy

There's always old, faithful walking as a means to maintain physical strength and endurance for women forty-five-plus. Brisk walking for just twenty to thirty minutes each day can be a metabolism booster (which we all need) and a secret to weight loss.

Walking is not just a good workout but can be a major factor in reducing the risk of developing disabling threats such as strokes, heart disease, certain cancers, osteoporosis, diabetes, and even depression. Walking each day can also strengthen your back and can also stimulate the thought process.

Aiming for five days a week of walking activity can significantly change your life and make you feel like your best self.

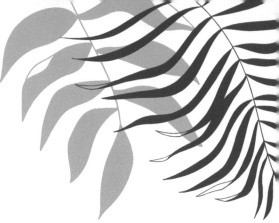

DANCE

"Dance is the hidden language of the soul." —*Martha Graham*

Have you ever watched the show *Dancing with the Stars* on TV and wondered, "I wish I could do that!" Just when you think it might be time to give up on learning the tango or the cha-cha or even the waltz, think again!

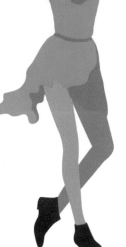

If you're having some back and hip issues, you may not want a partner swinging you around their neck, but ballroom dancing is a great way to achieve a healthier spine, and again, a strong core. Good posture and a strong back can be a key to maintaining health as we age and becoming the best versions of ourselves inside and out. Ballroom dancing typically has a low impact on the body and the motion can be beneficial to women with arthritis, stiff muscles, and joint pain.

Not to mention, dancing keeps the brain active and learning. For those who are high-risk for acquiring dementia, keeping the brain stimulated reduces the risk significantly. As always, consult with your doctor before signing up for a class.

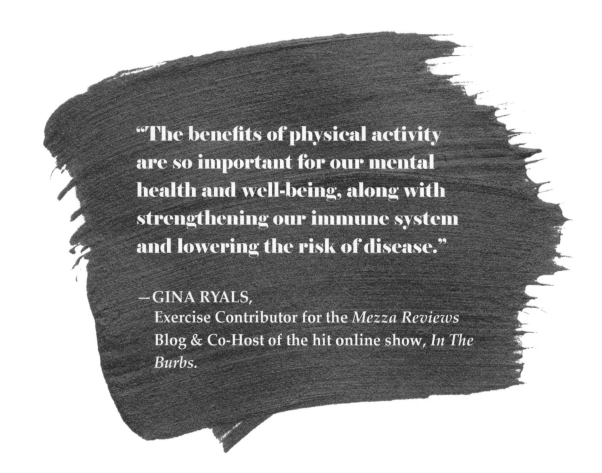

"The benefits of physical activity are so important for our mental health and well-being, along with strengthening our immune system and lowering the risk of disease."

—GINA RYALS,
Exercise Contributor for the *Mezza Reviews* Blog & Co-Host of the hit online show, *In The Burbs*.

PHYSICAL MANAGEMENT

My lifeline is my smartwatch! Not only is a smartwatch a good investment for your physical health, it can also be a great asset to your mental health. This can also serve as a vital part of your self-care routine. A smartwatch can give your mind and body just a little more love.

As women, we wear many hats and face many things in the world each day. Personalizing your smartwatch can not only cater to your physical needs but can also be a style statement as well.

Just as important as having a smartwatch is finding the right one to fit your needs. Whether you want all the bells and whistles or just something as simple as monitoring your heart rate at any given time, your smartwatch can say a lot about you and what's important to you.

Portion control is my new yoga mantra!

Healthier habits make all the difference in your overall health as we enter into the more seasoned version of life. Practicing something as simple as portion control can be a natural adjustment you can make that doesn't require too much effort.

As we get older, our metabolism becomes slower and women begin losing about half a pound of muscle per year, starting at age forty. This doesn't have to be a sign that your body is breaking down, but rather a message to start controlling how much you eat at any given time.

Downsizing your portions doesn't have to be all bad. The key is making each meal "count." Eating a healthy dose of fruits and veggies while keeping proteins lean keeps your nutritional values in check, and monitoring how much of these foods you're eating can be an eating plan you can grow to love.

Go for the fiber-rich foods and even start using a calorie counter to always make sure you're staying the course. While these methods may not be trendy, they are effective in keeping you around long enough to enjoy the better half of your life.

"My passion for the beauty industry started with a desire to see more high-quality, clean performance care products come to the marketplace. The mission statement for the company I now work for is just that, to get safe products into the hands of everyone."

—JUDY GOLDBERG,
   Clean Beauty Contributor for
   the *Mezza Reviews* blog.

SKIN HEALTH

One of the most telltale signs of age is our skin! Maintaining a healthy skin routine is vital for keeping yourself fresh and healthy. Your skin changes with age and we can't do much to slow down the process, however, the better care we take of our skin, the better our skin will be to us!

There are wonderful brands out there that can add collagen and keep you looking fresh and fabulous. My go-to for searching out new brands is to head over to your social media sites. You can order directly on these sites. Another thing you need to do is find a great dermatologist who is also making sure you are staying safe from too much sun exposure. I also like to visit my local spas for a fun facial, peel, or skin treatment monthly.

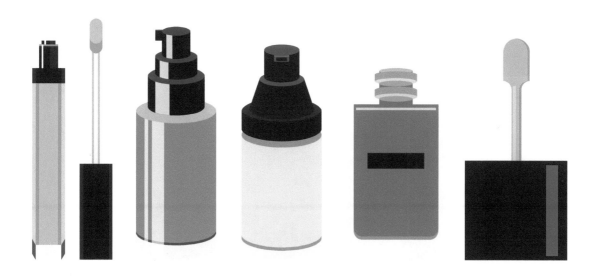

MICRODERM

Beautiful skin is a blessing, and you can still have it even in your fabulous forties, fifties, and beyond. Microdermabrasion has many benefits including:

- diminishing fine line and wrinkles

- reducing damaged skin and pores

- increasing circulation

- improving discoloration

- exfoliating skin

- reduction of acne scars

- a smoother skin surface

While your teenage skin may be in the past, you can still look great and healthy with noninvasive microdermabrasion treatments. It's all about finding which one will be the right fit for you.

DERMABLADING

In recent years, dermablading has become increasingly popular for all skin types. It consists of physical exfoliation using sterile, surgical scalpels to shave the top level of dead skin cells to prevent any hair on the face . . . or what we like to call "peach fuzz."

Sometimes, the more seasoned our skin gets, the more this peach fuzz begins to appear. Cellular regeneration starts to increasingly decline, and the skin begins to need more and more hydration. Trigger your regeneration and start making your skin age backward with your first treatment.

Please be advised that any dermablading should be done under the advisement of a licensed medical practitioner.

These are all practices that I follow.

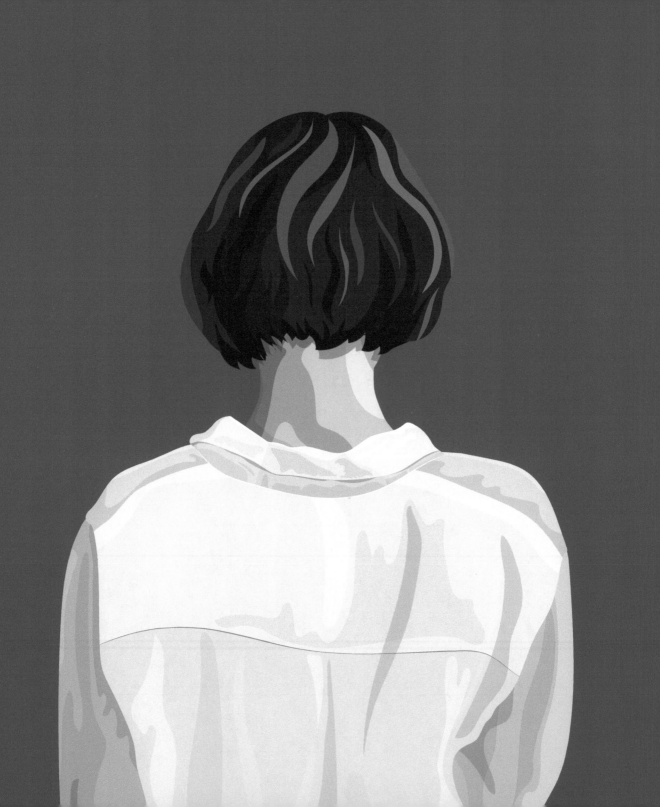

HEALTHY HAIR

With Insights from LaShena Spencer—Hairstylist

As we age, our hair changes. Everything from the texture, thickness, style, and, of course, color ages with us, meaning by the time you hit your early forties, you could be battling a completely different hair type than what you had in your twenties and thirties.

From split ends, frizziness, dryness, thinning, and (the most obvious one) gray strands, aging hair can be confusing and frustrating.

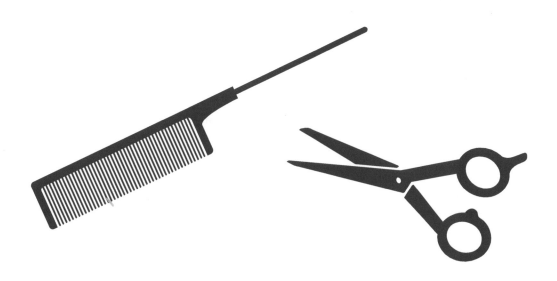

HAIR TIPS FOR WOMEN OVER FORTY-FIVE

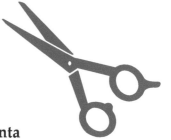

by LaShena Spencer—Hairstylist, Atlanta

- Eliminate the daily washes if you can help it, for it dries the hair out over time as we get older.

- Don't be afraid of going shorter or adding layers for more movement; keep up with trims routinely.

- Use extensions to give the illusion of thicker, fuller hair; this could vary on hair density/texture (tape ins, keratin tips, micro links, halo, etc.).

- Products are key! All hair types are not created equal.

- If you struggle using a round brush and a hairdryer, try using a product that incorporates both brush and hairdryer in one. A spinning round brush with a dryer built in is a great way to get instant volume.

- Hair treatments are also important. Twice a month, consider deep conditioning your hair, which will help your hair retain its moisture.

- Add color, balayage, or highlights. This can truly make a difference in a new look.

HAIR LOSS

It's almost as if, as soon as you hit forty-five, things start changing with your hair, including dryness, brittleness, thinning, and even being less manageable. All women should know that this is completely normal, and *you are not alone!*

Some of these changes can cause a slight loss of hair. The important thing to note is that these changes will happen slow and subtly.

Hormones play a huge part in hair loss. As women age, estrogen levels decline as they head toward menopause. If you are starting to feel these changes, consult with your doctor about supplements that could help and cue up a recipe for success.

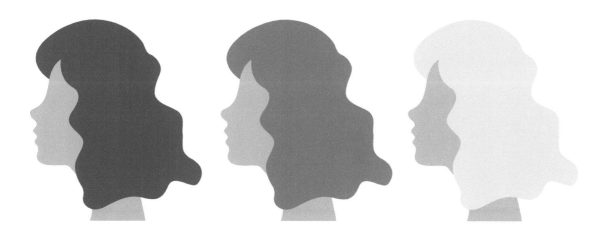

HEALTHY NAILS

W ho says you can't be fabulous with your nails after forty-five?

Your nails are your finishing touch to any look that you create. Your nails can really make your outfit complete, especially if you are like me and love to co-ordinate your nails with your outfits. Nails can express your creativity with your color choices, designs, shape, and even jewels to put on them.

MONTHLY NAIL CARE

The best way to keep your nails healthy and beautiful is to proceed with regular maintenance. Whether weekly, bi-weekly, or monthly, a good manicure or pedicure helps to develop your nails, especially as you age. We use our hands and feet every single day in some way or another, so it's ideal to keep them looking as young and fresh as possible.

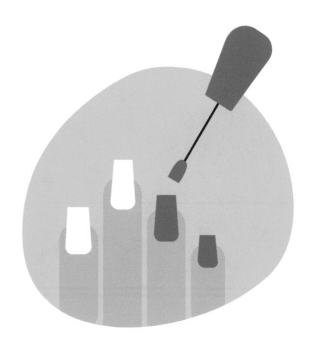

BIKINI MAINTENANCE

This is truly something I can't live without. No '70s look here! Bikini maintenance has no age limit! A nice wax, from a trusted and certified esthetician, can truly make a difference in how you act and feel.

Whichever waxing option you choose, whether bikini or Brazilian, your bikini maintenance habits can make you get your sexy back, or enhance it altogether. If you want a way that makes you feel right back in your twenties, this is the thing!

This can be a daunting task, but also a daring one. Your forties and fifties are for taking the risks you were too scared to take earlier in life. Be prepared for a little discomfort; however, a little discomfort can go a long way! Just remember that exfoliation is KEY! A simple sugar scrub before and after will keep you feeling smooth and comfortable throughout your waxing experience.

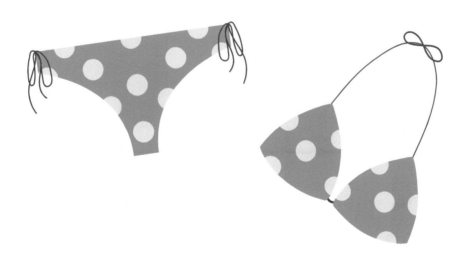

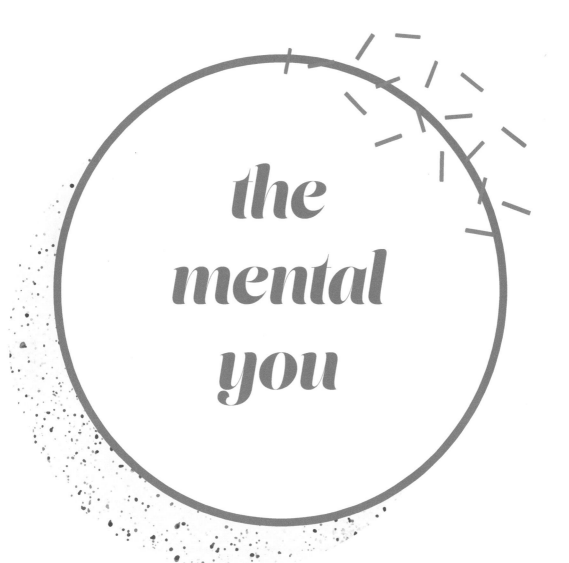

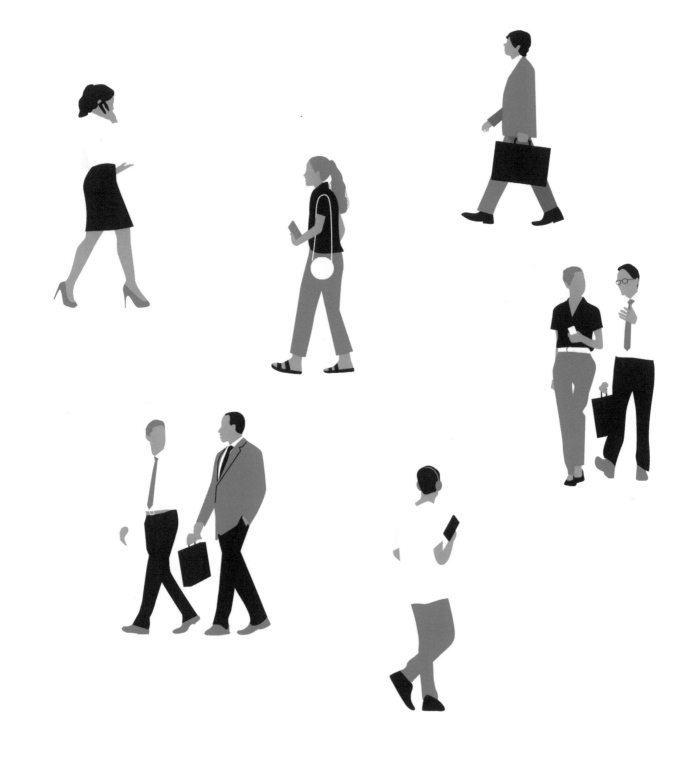

NETWORKING GROUPS

Many people believe that you should only network when looking for a new job or when you're young and on the hunt for your first big break. NEWS FLASH! Networking never stops. Networking groups that interest you can be so much fun and informative.

When considering joining networking groups, pick ones that add value to you and are of interest to you.

As an avid fashionista, I love to join fashion groups. The best thing about it is being surrounded by like-minded people who share my love for fashion and design. Since the pandemic, many networking groups have gone virtual. I do long for the day when we can all gather safely and in person.

I encourage you to join groups which interest you and are attended by people of like-minded interests as yourself. There's always a group of people out there, just like you, who share everything you value and more.

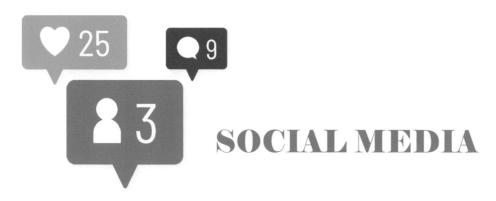

SOCIAL MEDIA

The world is social!

Back in 2000, who knew we would center our lives around social media? It has quickly become a way of life for many and an easy way to experience life updates from those we want to stay connected with.

For me, I enjoy all the platforms, not just for business but to stay current in our fast-paced society as a whole.

Not only does social media allow for us to stay connected, it also gives us the opportunity to follow people of influence based on our interest, age, and demographics. This is a great opportunity to also follow my blog, *Mezza Reviews*. We cover all the hot topics for us girls in the middle, like health, lifestyle, fashion, entertainment, home decor, and more. If you're into fashion, like I am, following fashion influencers who are over forty-five gives me great inspiration for my own personal style and lifestyle tips.

We're fortunate to have evolved enough in society to have a little bit of something for everyone.

Pro tip: Use your social media platforms like search engines. Explore new things and people that align with your life and pass along the information to others. This helps us expand our perspectives and experience things we might not otherwise know about.

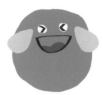

GET OUT OF YOUR COMFORT ZONE

Totally do this!

The times we are living in cause us to truly take stock in what we find fulfilling in our lives. If you find yourself stuck in a rut, it's time to start making some changes. It's easy to get caught up in the daily responsibilities of life, whether it's taking care of children, aging parents, spouses, the home, work, or more, finding time to explore new possibilities for yourself can keep you on a track to happiness.

I make it a habit to get out of my comfort zone often. When I started writing my blog, it was one of the first things I did for myself that pushed me out of my comfort zone and into a brand-new passion. This led to a number of other things I've been able to explore, including being a host on a live-stream, online show.

Another cool, new exploration is learning how to play mah jong. It's become a new craze among the tail end of the Baby Boomers and we should be here for it! The way I see it, if Sarah Jessica Parker is playing it, then I want in too!

One lesson I've learned with this is that having the courage to step out of your comfort zone can not only lead to new opportunities, but it can also help you to understand yourself better in a way that uncovers passions you may not have explored for a long time!

"Flowers are a love of mine. They bring me joy, and when I design a floral arrangement, my creativity and originality tend to flourish. I am the happiest when I have my hands in the soil. Planting flowers, shrubs, and landscaping provide me with peace and connectivity to the earth."

— ANNE VALGOI,
Floral & Entertaining Contributor for the *Mezza Reviews* blog.

NEW HOBBIES

Engaging in a new hobby is always a good idea!

When you get to this stage of life, you may find that you have more time than before. Your kids may be out of the house, or you may be reinventing your life, so finding a new hobby that you enjoy enough to spend an extended amount of time doing is important.

One thing that I've thought about taking up again as an old hobby is knitting. I also carve out time to work out, write, and spend time with my granddaughters. Wine tasting has always been a love of mine but actually making it a hobby to learn more about is still on my list. When the world gets back to what will be our new normal, I'd also love to get back my passion for travel.

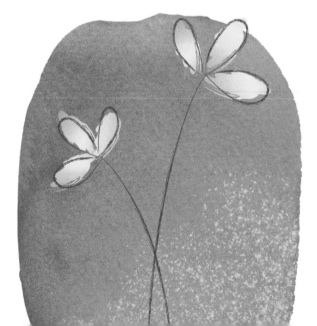

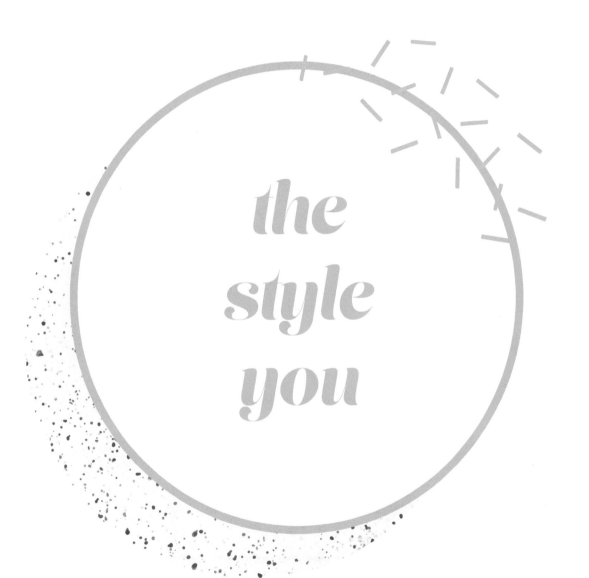

the
style
you

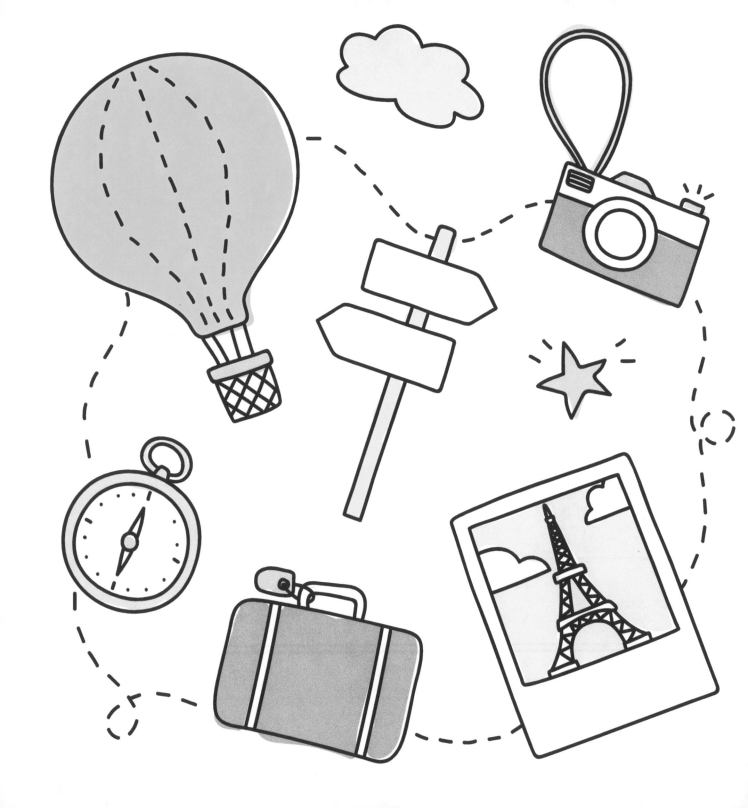

GET INSPIRATION

We can all use a little inspiration. Because we evolve so much during our lives, getting inspiration over the age of forty-five can get us to look at things differently and create perspectives that allow us to come into who we deserve to be.

There are many ways to get inspiration within your life:

- follow inspirational websites

- follow influencers

- join a networking group

- go on a trip

- talk with friends

- have time to yourself

- practice self-care

VISION BOARD

Getting ideas, looking up outfits, colors, and design can all be done by looking online as well as in magazines and catalogs, then you can make a vision board either online or through cutting out pictures—old school but it works. A great way to reference outfits that you may want to remember!

FOLLOW BRANDS

One of the most important things about getting inspired is ensuring that there is no age limitation to what you explore. When it comes to brands, there can be a stigma attached to specific ones. We believe that although there are brands who cater to women between the ages of forty-five and beyond, we shouldn't be limited to that in order to gain style inspiration.

Following brands—whether through social media channels, blogs, or frequent website visits—can help in gauging your own personal evolution.

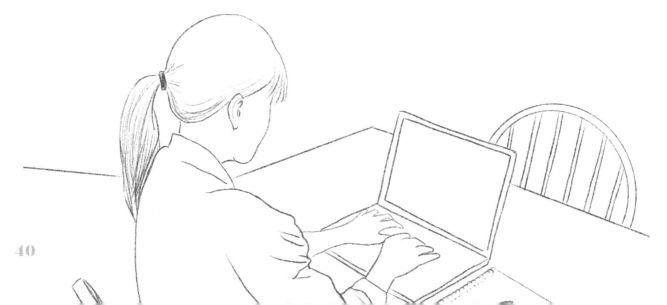

THE ART OF STYLE

Look at each outfit you wear as a piece of art and make sure it's pleasing to you and has balance. Example, you don't want to wear too many colors or have too much jewelry on or even too many patterns. Always give yourself that final edit and approval.

SHOP YOUR CLOSET

Shopping doesn't just have to happen in the stores. You can find new and innovative items sitting right there in your closet.

One way to help you shop in your closet is by making a big purge. Purging can consist of getting rid of items that no longer fit you, are out of style, or may just not be your personal style anymore. Keeping these items can create clutter for your closet and can even cloud your overall judgement of what you like and what you don't. When you purge, you create space for new and fresh items that can be added to your collection.

Part of being able to shop your closet means you first have to have the right items in it that make sense for your evolving style.

When you begin to shop your closet, you are able to use your creativity in a new way to develop outfits that you might have never chosen before.

STAPLE ITEMS

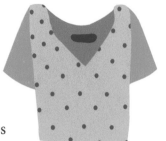

- long and short blazers

- a cardigan sweater

- scarves

- belts

- statement shoes

- boots (tall, short, cowboy)

- flats (ballet and loafer slides)

- sandals and mules

- dress shoes (open- or closed-toe heels)

- bags & purses (evening, straw, and totes)

- white blouses

- printed blouses

- skirts

- leggings

- trench coats

- little black dresses

- denim jeans

- white jeans

- black slacks

- palazzo pants

- cropped pants

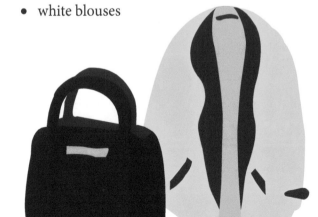

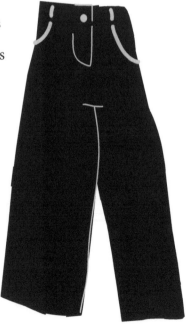

UNDERGARMENTS

Undergarments become so much more important the older you get! Now, there are unspoken rules that we have to follow in order to make sure everything stays intact and smooth.

Here are some dos and don'ts of undergarments:

- **DON'T** wear bras that you dug out of your drawer from the previous two presidential administrations, or before the internet.

- **DO** get bra fittings at least once a year to avoid the "girls" from dragging on the floor. A no-surgery lift is always a good thing.

- **DO** get good, quality shapewear that you can wear under a dress or slacks for a smoother appearance. This is the key to getting a tummy tuck or liposuction without going under the knife.

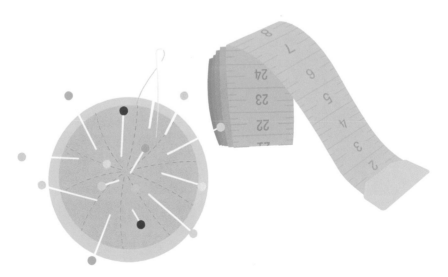

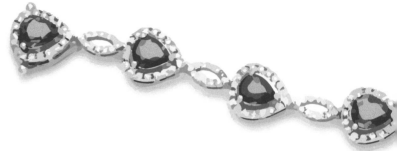

STATEMENT JEWELRY

Owning your jewelry style is all about what makes you feel the most comfortable.

A good statement piece can increase your self-esteem and make you look and feel more confident. However, there is a limit as to what kind of statement you want to make as someone in their forties and beyond.

During this stage of life, it's all about balance and knowing what you want to accentuate on your body and what you don't. By this age, we are well-versed as to what our best body parts are, as well as what areas we tend to want to hide from others. Finding jewelry that can enhance the parts of us we like can make you feel great in every way.

This is the time to play up your creativity. A plain outfit can be made to be more interesting with a formal piece of jewelry that packs a punch. Have fun with it and try different things. Experiment with different metals and jewels. See what colors work with you and what does not. My only request is that you keep it simple and not too match-y.

TRENDING ITEMS AND WAYS TO WEAR

When we reach middle age, instead of following all the trends, it's best to pick an accessory that reflects the trend of the season and stick with that.

The things that are best to leave to the twenty-year-olds are rompers, short skirts, and shorts! Instead, try a great pencil skirt or an A-line skirt that can show off your figure and still keep you feeling confident.

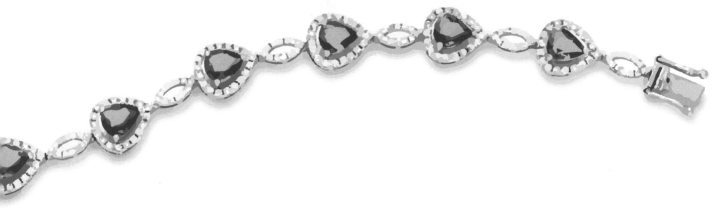

Another DON'T for us middle-aged women are harem pants and some joggers. We don't want to relive the worst of the seventies. Go for palazzo pants instead. They keep your waist cinched while still giving a wide-leg appeal.

When we get to this age, we also want to avoid the muffin top at all costs. Low-rise jeans and slacks paired with short knit shirts are a recipe for the ultimate muffin top. What you can wear as an alternative to a casual, laid-back look are jeans and slacks that hit you right below the belly button. Currently, high-waisted jeans are in, but beware of the mom jeans from the eighties that are seemingly trying to make a comeback with Generation Z.

When looking at dresses, the iconic Diane Von Furstenburg wrap dress will always remain a classic. Trust me, your daughter will thank you for letting go of the micro mini you were wearing in the sixties—unless you were asked to be in the next Austin Powers movie.

When it comes to color, try not to always hide behind black. It's so easy to make this your go-to color, especially when trying to hide our problem areas, but let's brighten our forty-five-plus complexions. We didn't do all that skin care to only keep black as the staple color in our lives.

There is a secret to a sagging neck: grab a neck scarf! A great neck scarf will hide what you want and be fashionable at the same time.

Lastly, tailoring is in!

Small, medium, and large sizing are not always your friends. Your real buddy is your local tailor or dressmaker. Tailoring your garments is what makes your clothing fit you, instead of how your garments fit the masses. This is a regular practice for most men, but for women, the idea of tailoring can take a bit of convincing.

WHAT MAKES YOU BUY CLOTHES AT FORTY-FIVE-PLUS

I buy clothing every season because I want to not only add to my wardrobe but feel the need to have at least one or two pieces from the runways. Women who are forty-five-plus are still out here making money while holding down their careers and still wanting to keep themselves relevant and sexy, yet not looking like they are trying too hard. You want to always STAND OUT, not STICK OUT.

Another reason I buy clothing each season is for travel. I perk up my travel wardrobe with a few key pieces:

- a great white shirt

- a new travel wrap

- good walking shoes

- black dress/skirt that won't wrinkle

Being invited to a black-tie event is another great reason to shop. I recently found that small, boutique wedding shops have a wonderful display of after-five, short and long dresses. They are not just for the mother of the bride or groom. Here are some tips for buying after-five dresses:

Tip 1: if traveling to an event by plane, bring a second dress in case your first one has a malfunction, or someone comes in with the same outfit.

Tip 2: buy two pieces to avoid seeing yourself coming and going. For example, a long or short skirt and a top or sweater, depending on the season.

Tip 3: if you are the mother of the bride or groom, have someone tweak your outfit by adding a special design, which has meaning to you.

Finally, I love to shop to change my mood. There is nothing that compares to a little retail therapy, except a glass of wine with your significant other!

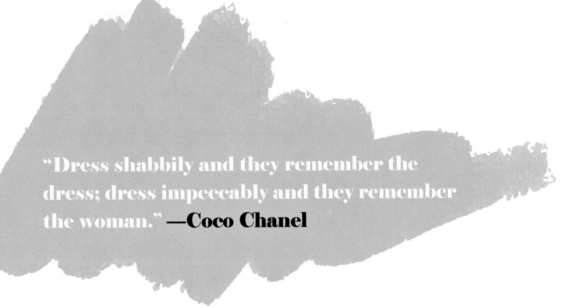

"Dress shabbily and they remember the dress; dress impeccably and they remember the woman." —**Coco Chanel**

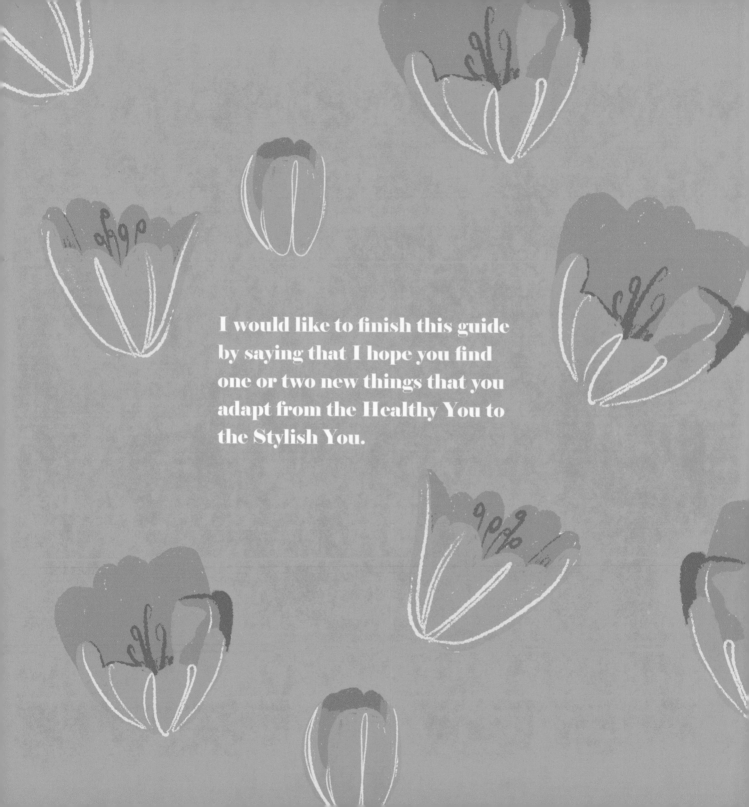

I would like to finish this guide by saying that I hope you find one or two new things that you adapt from the Healthy You to the Stylish You.

ACKNOWLEDGMENTS

I would like to give a special thanks to all the writers and contributors that make up the *Mezza Reviews* lifestyle blog.

Thank you

ABOUT JACQUELINE
FASHION/LIFESTYLE EXPERT

Jacqueline Grund is a fashion and lifestyle expert with a passion for uplifting women to be the best versions of themselves. She has had over twenty-five years of experience in fashion and the women's apparel industry. Her experience as a personal shopper for a high-end clothing store and as a personal stylist has lent to her overall mission of empowering women to step into the most authentic versions of themselves while feeling their best doing it.

She believes that style does not just stop when you turn forty-five but just begins in a new and different way! She continues to empower other women through her ambassadorship with many brands while bringing other women together to shop and feel good. She further promotes her mission through her successful lifestyle blog, *Mezza Reviews*, and her newly developed online show, *The MEZZA Live*, now seen @mezzagirl1959 or past shows on social media where she highlights fashion brands, style tips, travel recommendations, and home decor ideas for all women over forty-five.

For more information on Jacqueline, please visit www.MezzaReviews.com.

CPSIA information can be obtained
at www.ICGtesting.com
Printed in the USA
LVHW071917141021
700448LV00001B/17